DIFFUSER BLENDS *for* EVERYDAY

SIMPLYREENI.COM

FIND ME ON INSTAGRAM: @SIMPLY_REENI

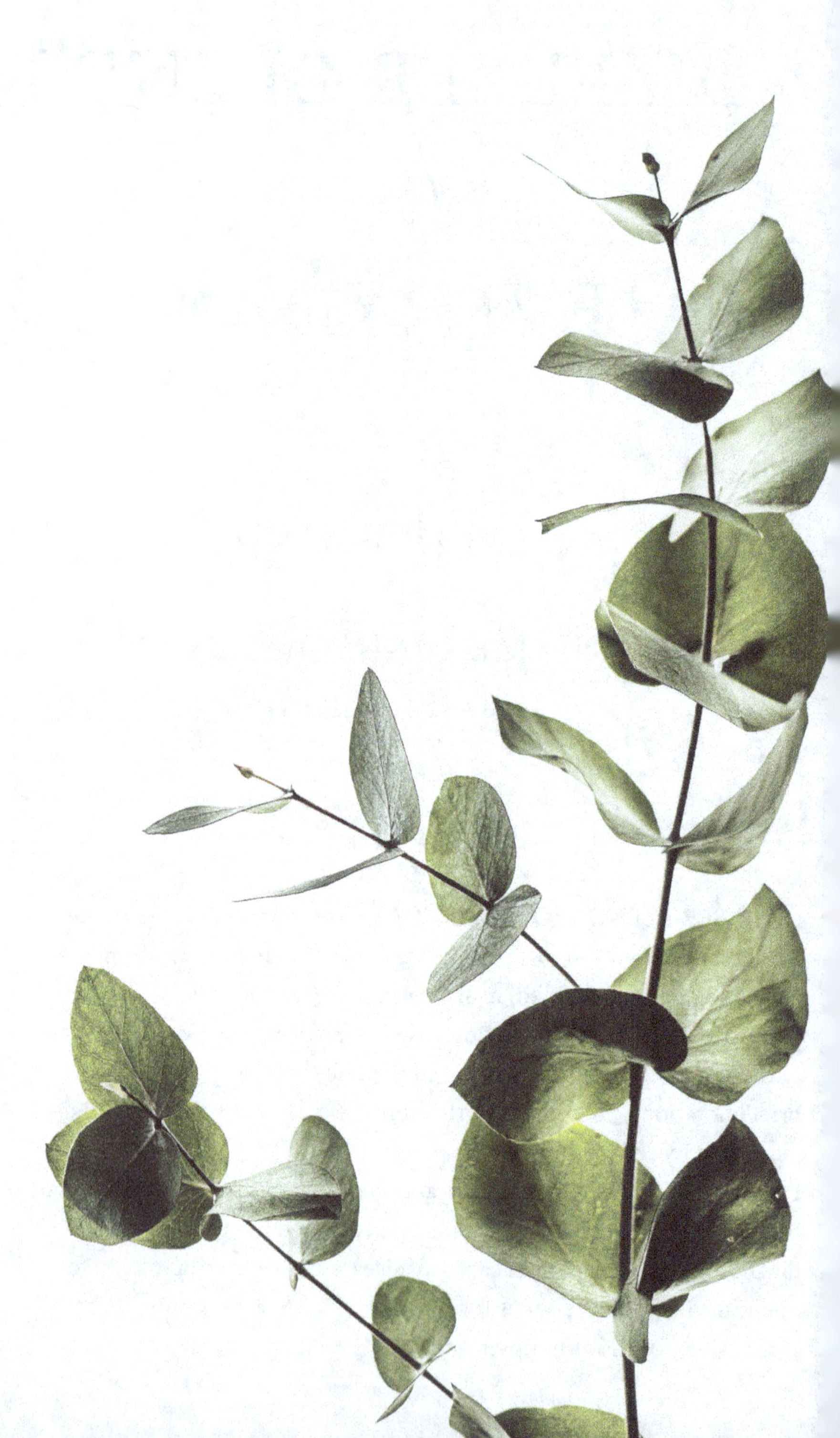

TABLE OF CONTENTS:

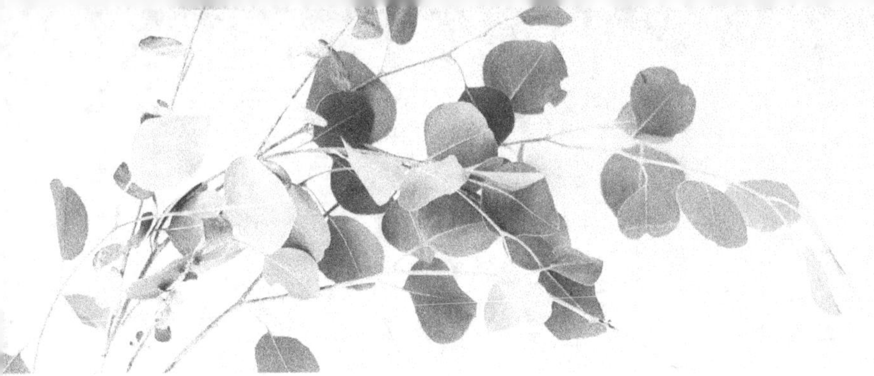

wake up

3 DROPS BASIL
3 DROPS LEMON

sunrise

2 DROPS TANGERINE
2 DROPS BERGAMOT
2 DROPS WILD ORANGE

rise

3 DROPS WILD ORANGE
2 DROPS PEPPERMINT
2 DROPS BERGAMOT

start the day

2 DROPS ROSEMARY
2 DROPS LEMON
2 DROPS TANGERINE

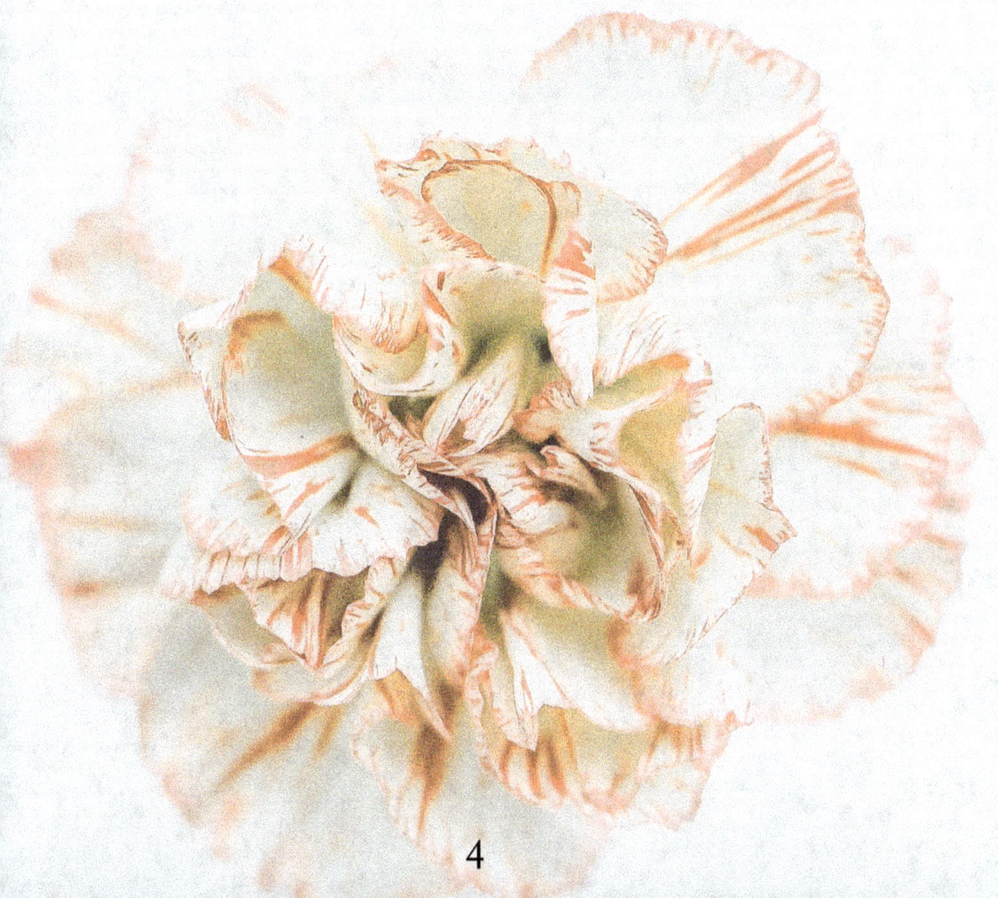

good morning

4 DROPS LEMON
3 DROPS PEPPERMINT

morning

2 DROPS WILD ORANGE
2 DROPS CINNAMON BARK
2 DROPS GINGER

rise and shine

3 DROPS PEPPERMINT
3 DROPS WILD ORANGE

calm morning

2 DROPS WILD ORANGE
2 DROPS VETIVER
2 DROPS FRANKINCENSE

start the day

2 DROPS ROSEMARY
2 DROPS WILD ORANGE
2 DROPS GRAPEFRUIT

energizing DIFFUSER BLENDS

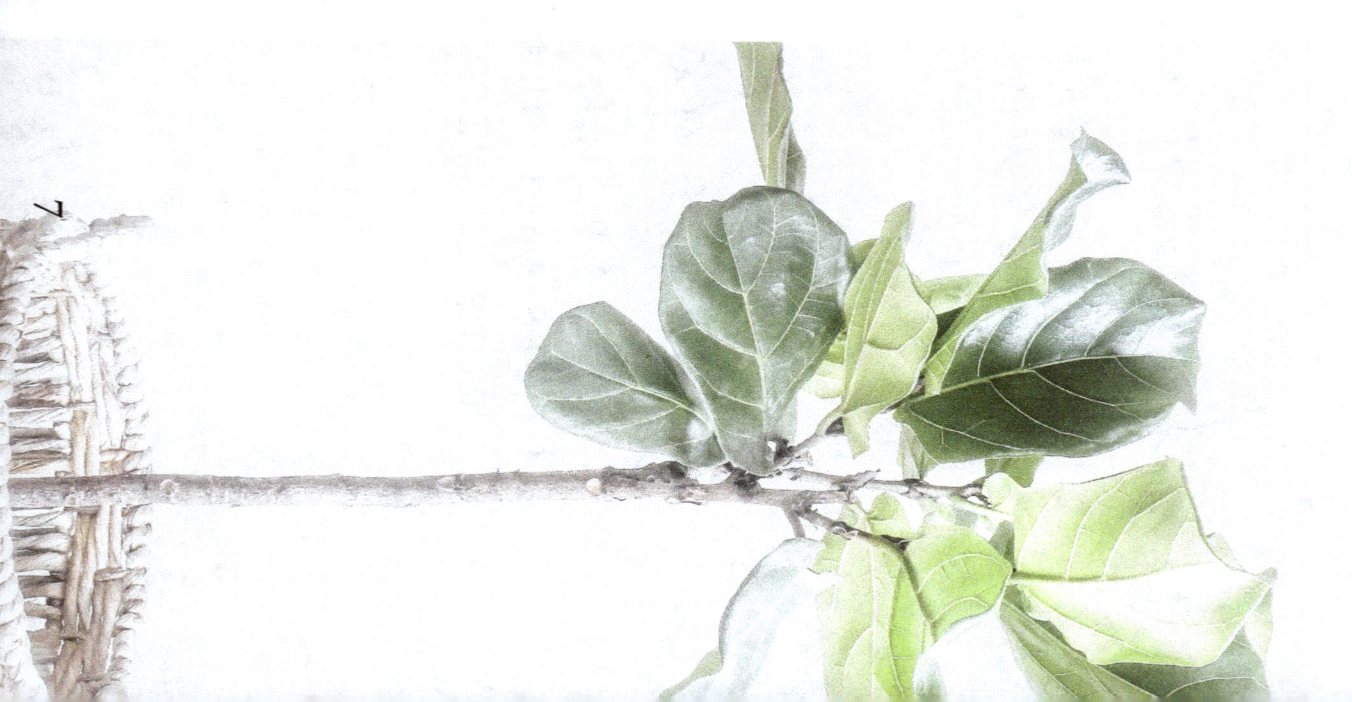

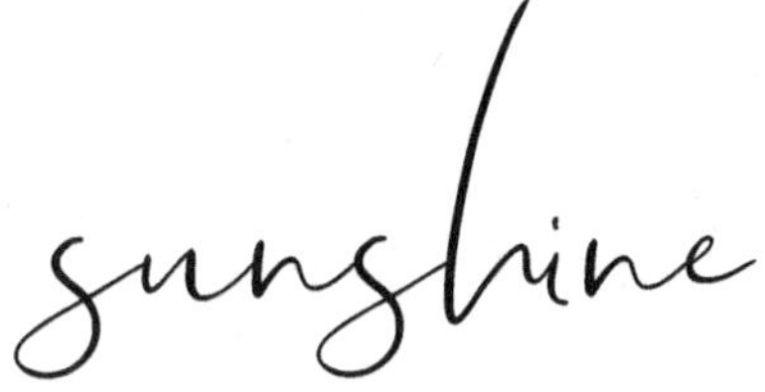

sunshine

3 DROPS PEPPERMINT
3 DROPS WILD ORANGE
3 DROPS TANGERINE

refresh

2 DROPS BERGAMOT
1 DROP CEDARWOOD
2 DROPS WINTERGREEN

focus & energize

3 DROPS GRAPEFRUIT
2 DROPS ROSEMARY
2 DROPS EUCALYPTUS

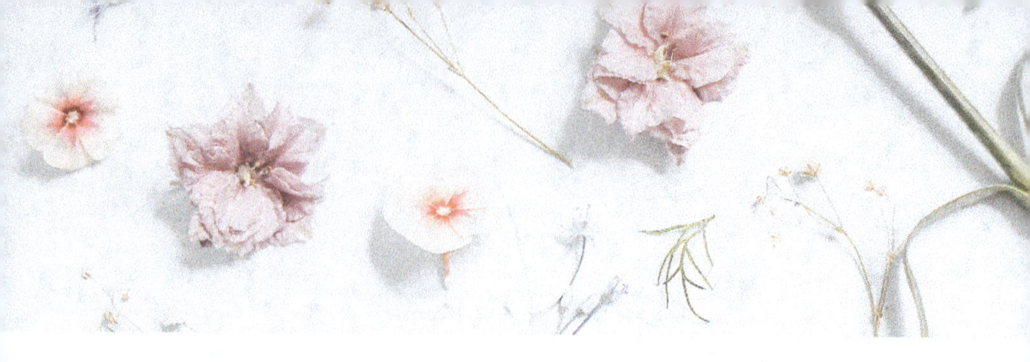

happy

2 DROPS BERGAMOT
2 DROPS SPEARMINT
2 DROPS TANGERINE

motivate

2 DROPS SPEARMINT
2 DROPS LEMON
2 DROPS WILD ORANGE

you can do it

2 DROPS JUNIPER BERRY
2 DROPS LIME
2 DROPS BERGAMOT

getting things done

1 DROP LEMON
2 DROPS ROSEMARY
2 DROPS WILD ORANGE
1 DROP PEPPERMINT

energizing

2 DROPS PEPPERMINT
2 DROPS LEMON
2 DROPS FRANKINCENSE

let's go

3 DROPS ROSEMARY
2 DROPS PEPPERMINT
2 DROPS BASIL

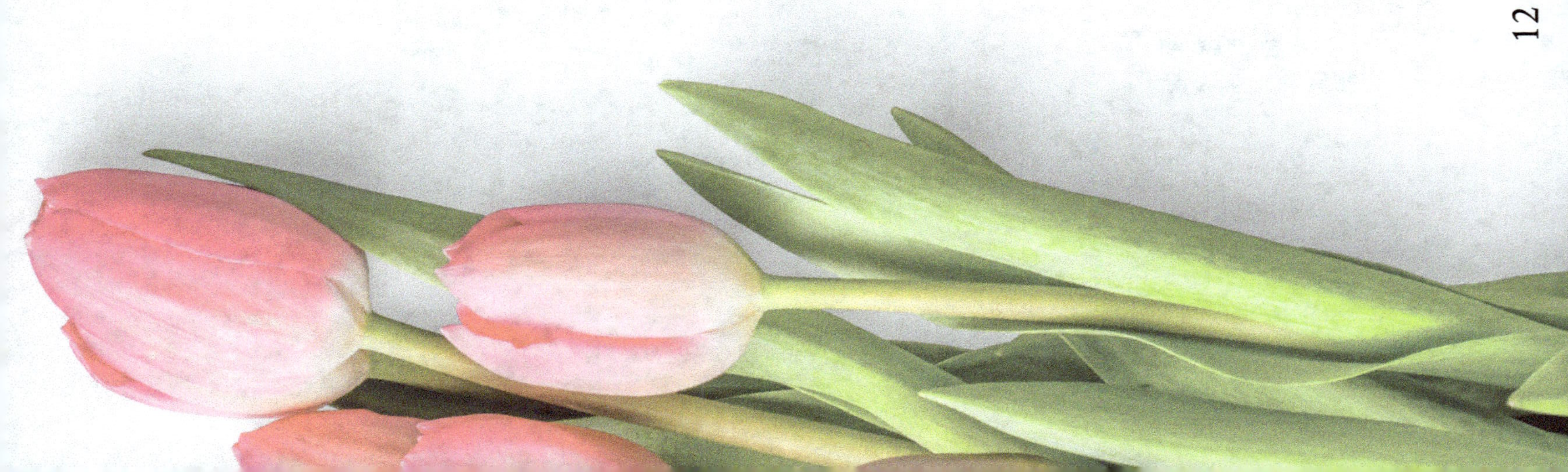

stress DIFFUSER BLENDS

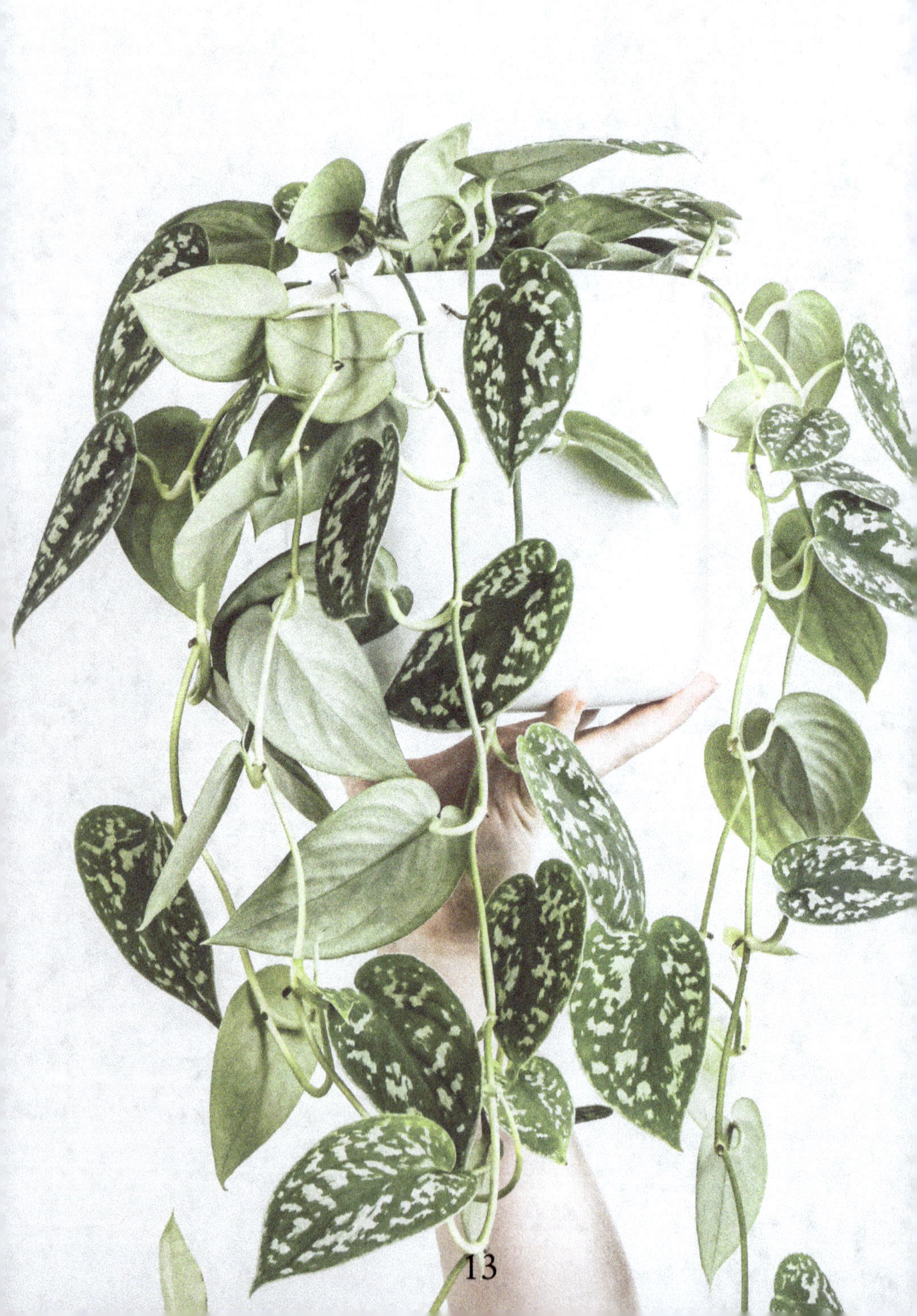

be still

3 DROPS LAVENDER
2 DROPS LIME
2 DROPS COPAIBA

breathe

2 DROPS ROMAN CHAMOMILE
2 DROPS LAVENDER
2 DROPS WILD ORANGE

evening bliss

2 DROPS CEDARWOOD
2 DROPS LAVENDER
2 DROPS COPAIBA

quiet time

3 DROPS ROMAN CHAMOMILE
3 DROPS LAVENDER

relax

3 DROPS LAVENDER
3 DROPS YLANG YLANG

stress less

2 DROPS FRANKINCENSE
2 DROPS LAVENDER
2 DROPS COPAIBA

rejuvenate

3 DROPS WILD ORANGE
3 DROPS LAVENDER

enjoy more

2 DROPS FRANKINCENSE
2 DROPS SIBERIAN FIR
2 DROPS CEDARWOOD

office DIFFUSER BLENDS

stay focused

2 DROPS ROSEMARY
2 DROPS PEPPERMINT
2 DROPS WILD ORANGE

start your day

2 DROPS PEPPERMINT
2 DROPS WILD ORANGE
2 DROPS BERGAMOT

stress less

3 DROPS LAVENDER
2 DROPS WILD ORANGE
1 DROP FRANKINCENSE

energize

3 DROPS BASIL
3 DROPS LEMON

long day

2 DROPS LAVENDER
2 DROPS ROSEMARY
2 DROPS LEMON

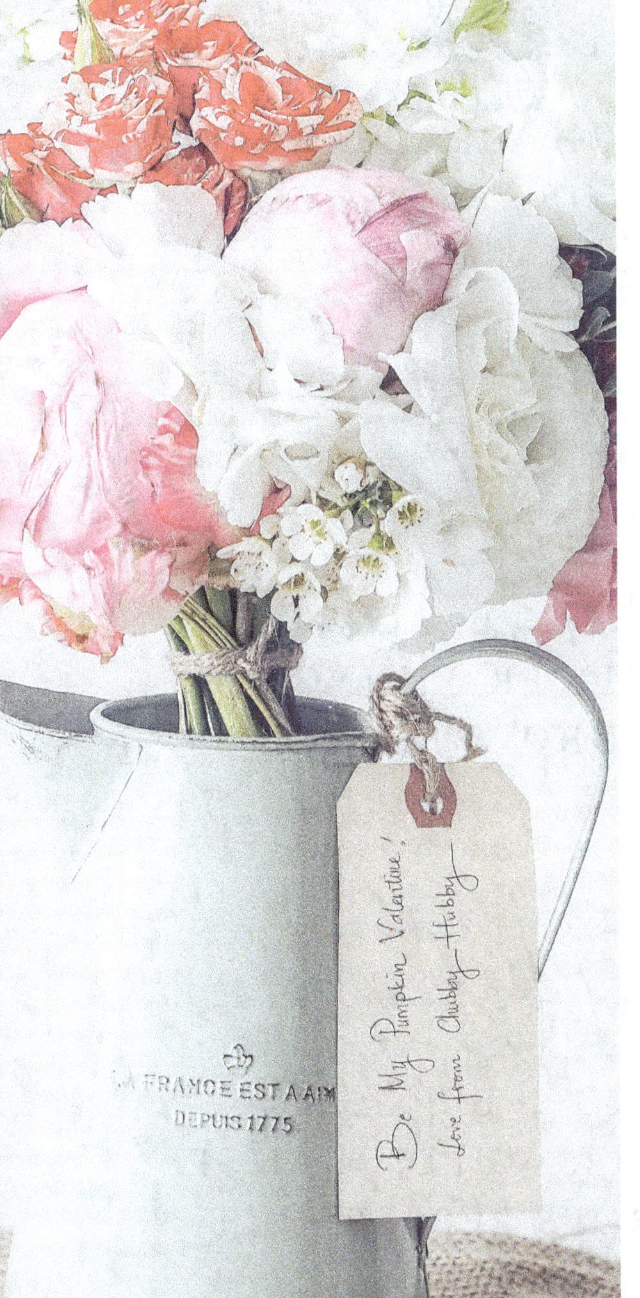

joyful

DIFFUSER BLENDS

joyful family

2 DROPS GRAPEFRUIT
2 DROPS BERGAMOT
2 DROPS WILD ORANGE

joyful

2 DROPS BERGAMOT
2 DROPS FRANKINCENSE
2 DROPS LEMON

uplifting

3 DROPS BERGAMOT
2 DROPS WILD ORANGE
2 DROPS PEPPERMINT

citrus bliss

2 DROPS LAVENDER
3 DROPS TANGERINE
3 DROPS WILD ORANGE

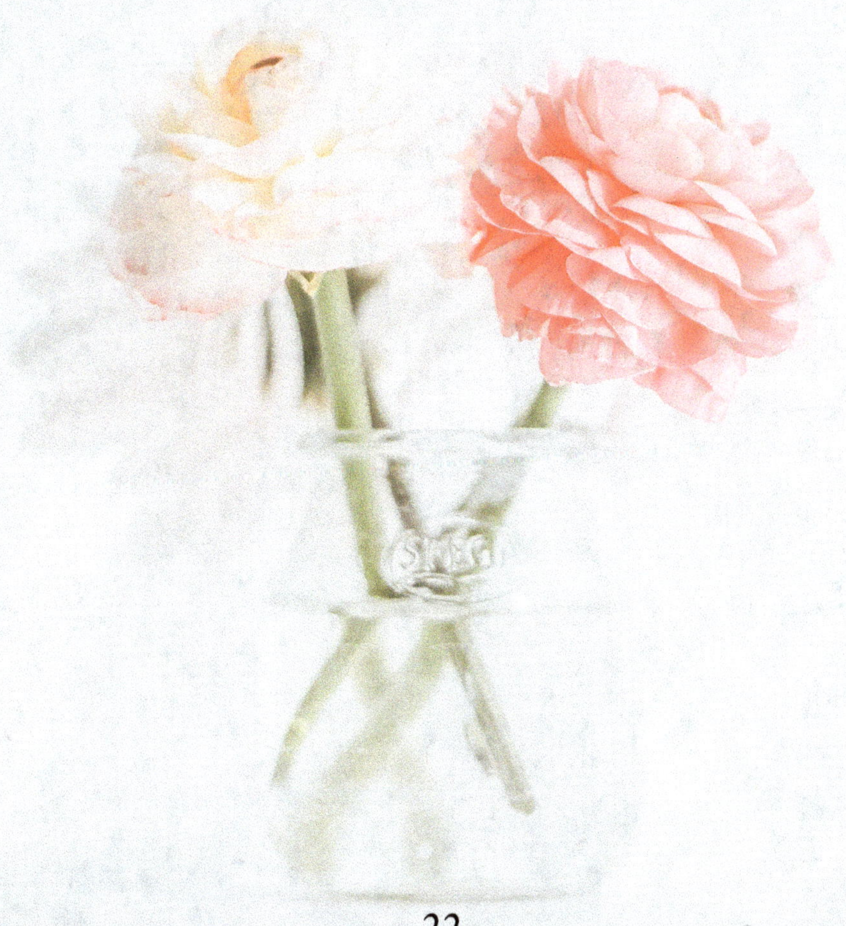

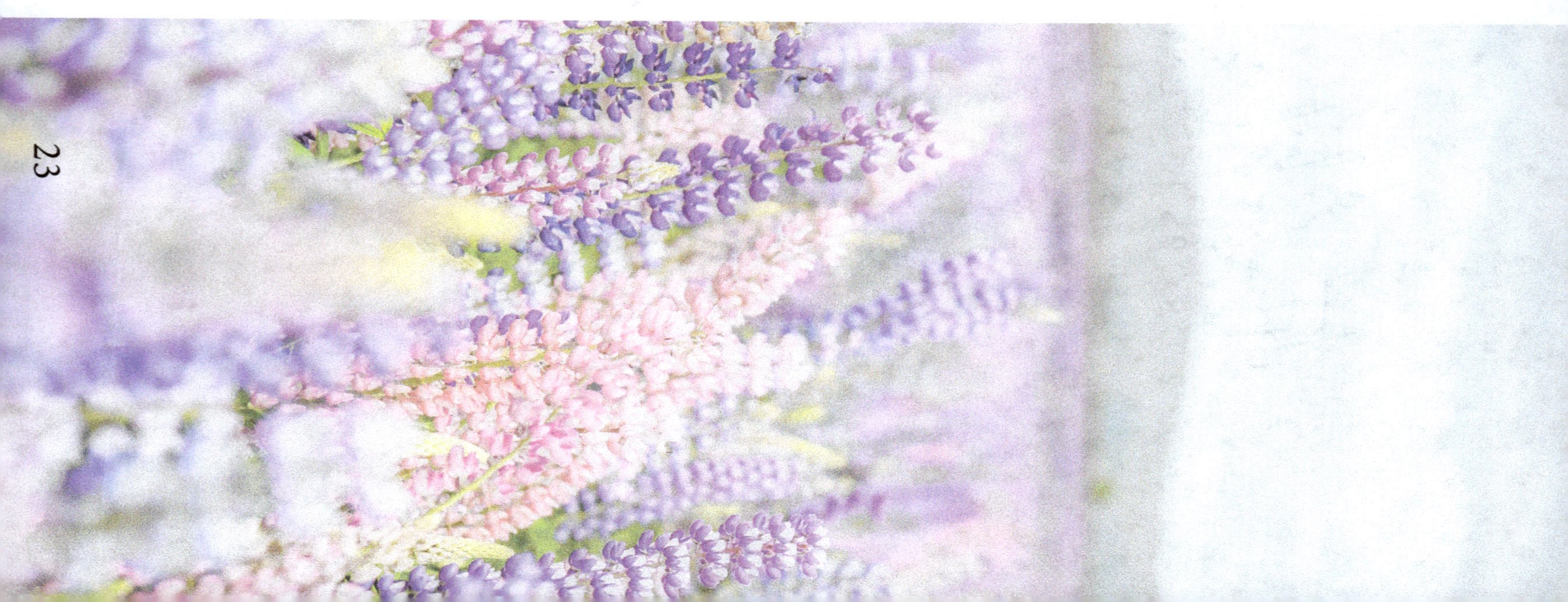

peaceful DIFFUSER BLENDS

beautiful life

3 DROPS YLANG YLANG
2 DROPS GERANIUM
2 DROPS CLARY SAGE

peaceful

3 DROPS VETIVER
2 DROPS LAVENDER
2 DROPS YLANG YLANG

relax

3 DROPS LAVENDER
3 DROPS CYPRESS
2 DROPS YLANG YLANG

immune

2 DROPS CLOVE
2 DROPS WILD ORANGE
1 DROP CINNAMON BARK

seasonal discomfort

2 DROPS LEMON
2 DROPS PEPPERMINT
2 DROPS LAVENDER

cleansing

3 DROPS LEMON
3 DROPS TEA TREE

respiratory support

2 DROPS EUCALYPTUS
2 DROPS CARDAMOM
2 DROPS LEMON

clean air

3 DROPS LAVENDER
3 DROPS LEMON

grounding

3 DROPS LAVENDER
2 DROPS CEDARWOOD
2 DROPS FRANKINCENSE
1 DROP VETIVER

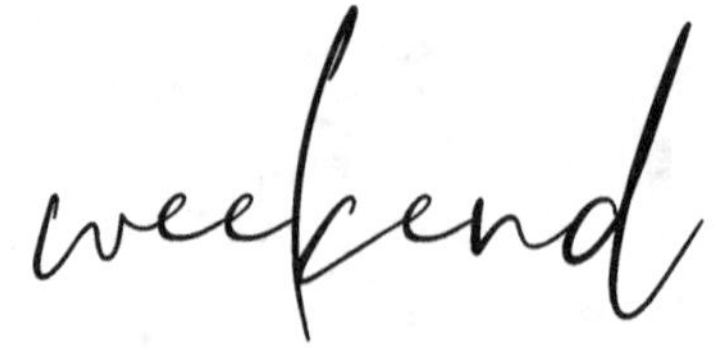

weekend

2 DROPS WILD ORANGE
3 DROPS BERGAMOT
2 DROPS FRANKINCENSE

calm evenings

3 DROPS LAVENDER
2 DROPS WILD ORANGE
1 DROP FRANKINCENSE

sunset

3 DROPS LAVENDER
3 DROPS CEDARWOOD

relaxation

2 DROPS VETIVER
2 DROPS FRANKINCENSE
2 DROPS LAVENDER

grounding

3 DROPS FRANKINCENSE
3 DROPS CEDARWOOD

calm mood

3 DROPS YLANG YLANG
2 DROPS WILD ORANGE
2 DROPS LAVENDER

dreamy

3 DROPS PATCHOULI
2 DROPS CYPRESS
2 DROPS BERGAMOT

soothing

3 DROPS LAVENDER
2 DROPS PATCHOULI
1 DROP YLANG YLANG

flowery

3 DROPS LAVENDER
2 DROPS JASMINE

love

3 DROPS BERGAMOT
2 DROPS PATCHOULI
2 DROPS YLANG YLANG

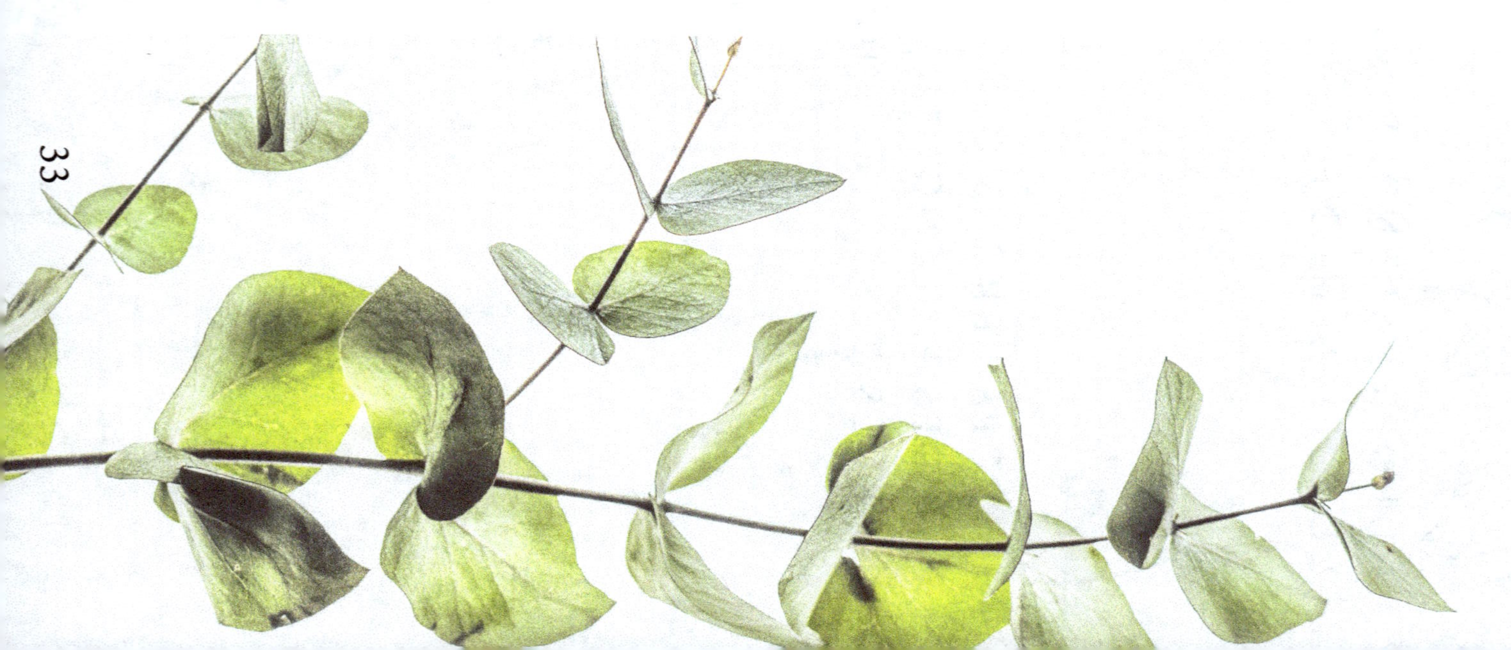

sleep DIFFUSER BLENDS

sleepy

2 DROPS VETIVER
2 DROPS CEDARWOOD
2 DROPS LAVENDER

goodnight

2 DROPS LAVENDER
3 DROPS ROMAN CHAMOMILE
1 DROP FRANKINCENSE

calm night

3 DROPS CEDARWOOD
3 DROPS LAVENDER

simple night

3 DROPS ROMAN CHAMOMILE
2 DROPS FRANKINCENSE
1 DROP VETIVER

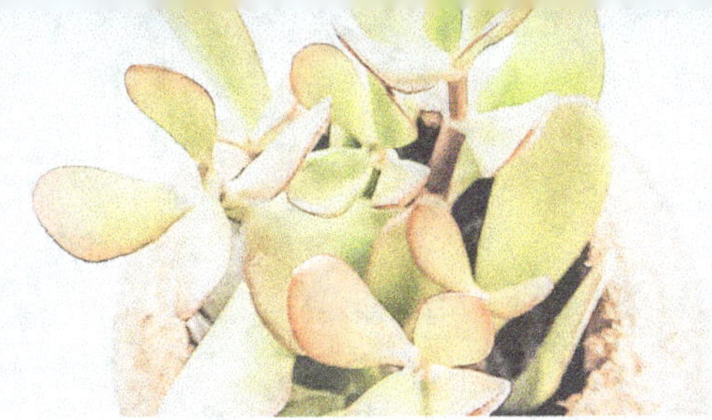

nighttime

3 DROPS LAVENDER
2 DROPS WILD ORANGE
2 DROPS SANDALWOOD

serene

3 DROPS YLANG YLANG
3 DROPS LAVENDER

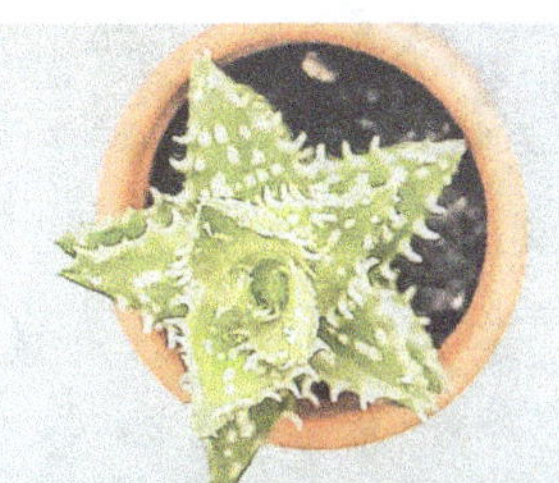

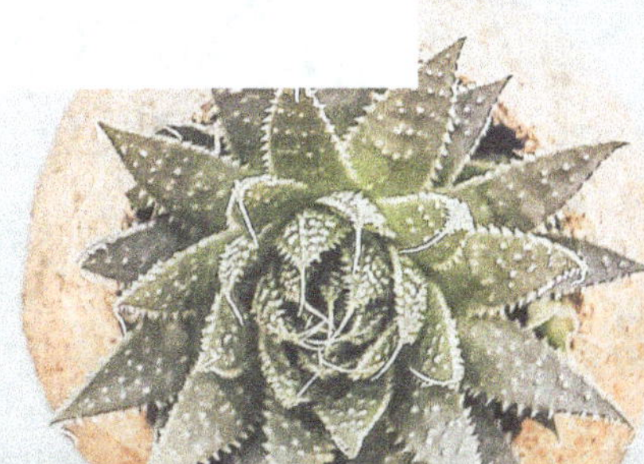

sweet dreams

3 DROPS JUNIPER BERRY
2 DROPS WILD ORANGE
2 DROPS GERANIUM

bedtime bliss

3 DROPS LAVENDER
3 DROPS BERGAMOT

dream

3 DROPS LAVENDER
2 DROPS CEDARWOOD
2 DROPS WILD ORANGE

fall DIFFUSER BLENDS

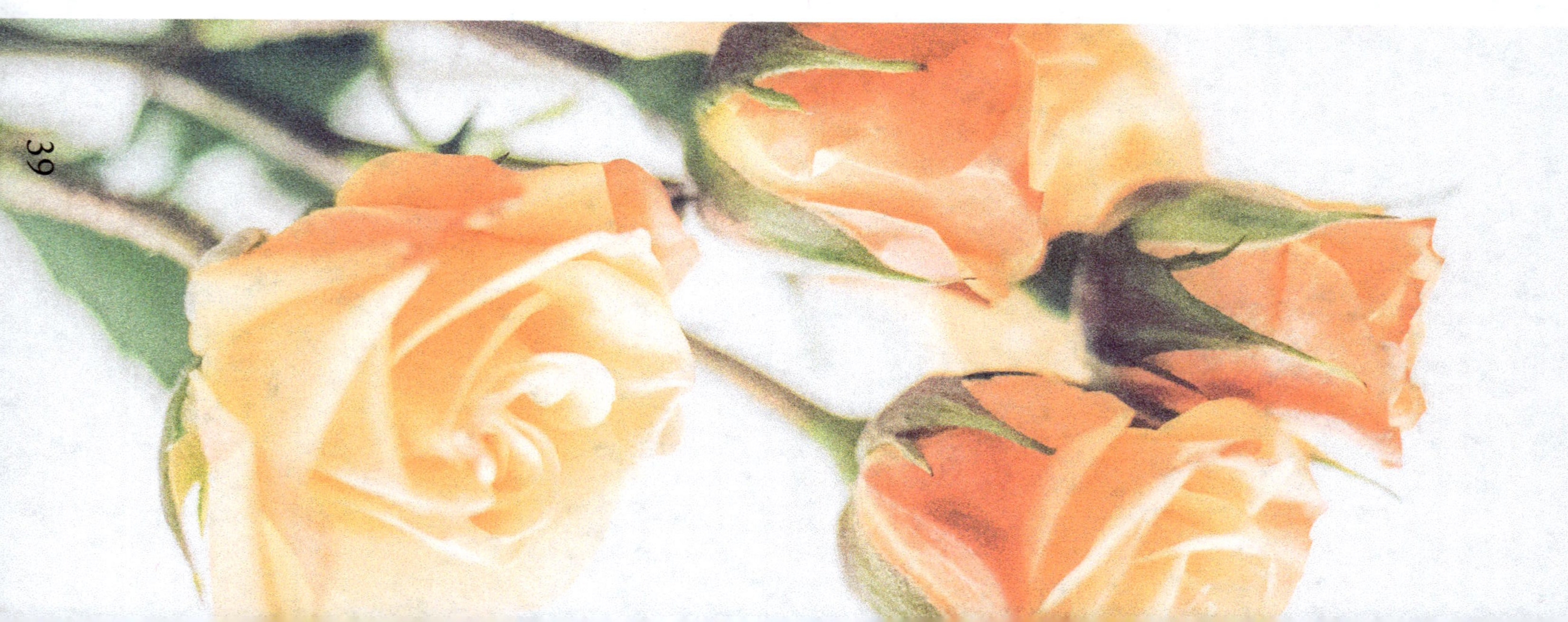

fall leaves

3 DROPS WILD ORANGE
2 DROPS CASSIA
2 DROPS CEDARWOOD

apple pie

2 DROPS DOUGLAS FIR
2 DROPS CINNAMON BARK
2 DROPS WILD ORANGE

cool breeze

2 DROPS LEMON
2 DROPS CARDAMOM
2 DROPS CASSIA

pumpkin spice

2 DROPS CINNAMON BARK
2 DROPS WILD ORANGE
2 DROPS CLOVE

fall spice

2 DROPS WILD ORANGE
2 DROPS CINNAMON BARK
2 DROPS GINGER

citrus fall

3 DROPS WILD ORANGE
2 DROPS BERGAMOT
1 DROP CINNAMON BARK

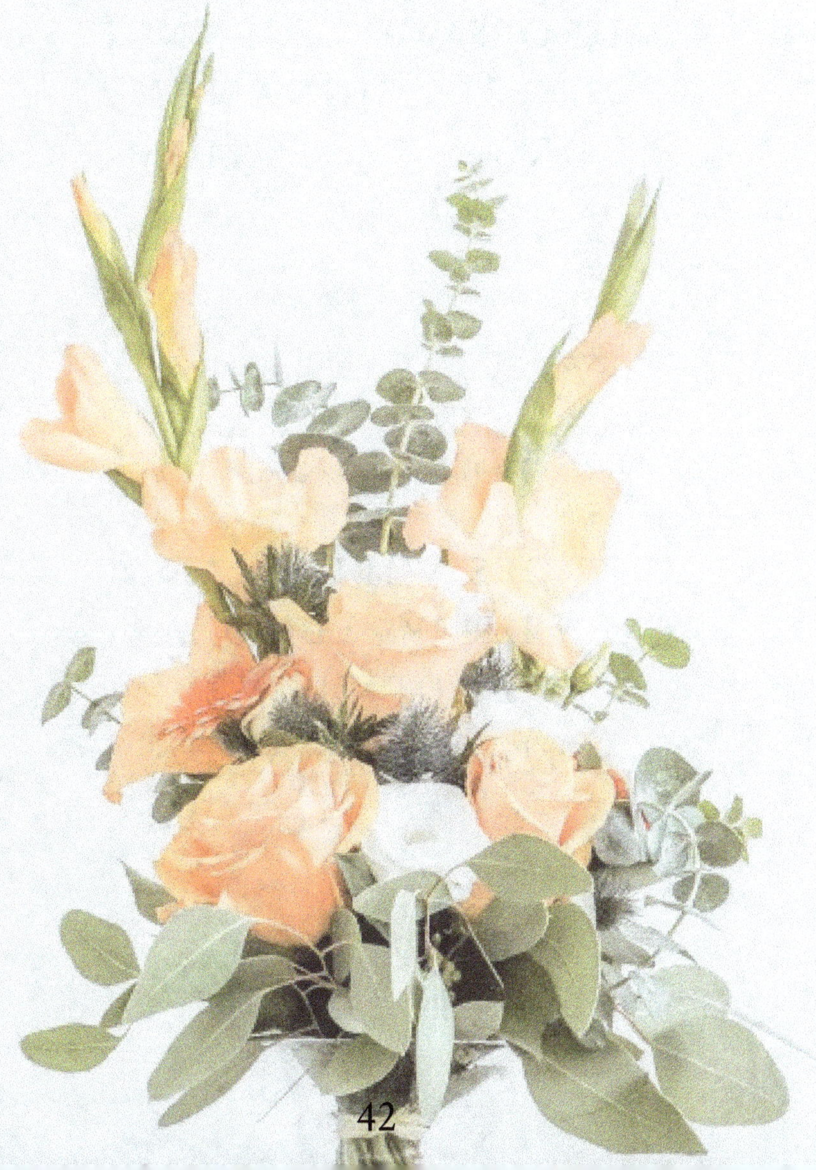

orange bliss

3 DROPS WILD ORANGE
2 DROPS CINNAMON
2 DROPS CARDAMOM

autumn

2 DROPS WILD ORANGE
2 DROPS LEMON
1 DROP CLOVE
1 DROP CINNAMON

2 DROPS CINNAMON BARK
2 DROPS WILD ORANGE
2 DROPS CLOVE

2 DROPS WILD ORANGE
2 DROPS BERGAMOT
2 DROPS PEPPERMINT

2 DROPS CEDARWOOD
2 DROPS SIBERIAN FIR
2 DROPS WILD ORANGE

2 DROPS LEMON
2 DROPS FRANKINCENSE
2 DROPS DOUGLAS FIR

uplifting

2 DROPS BERGAMOT
2 DROPS PEPPERMINT
2 DROPS FRANKINCENSE

snow day

2 DROPS LAVENDER
2 DROPS FRANKINCENSE
2 DROPS LEMON

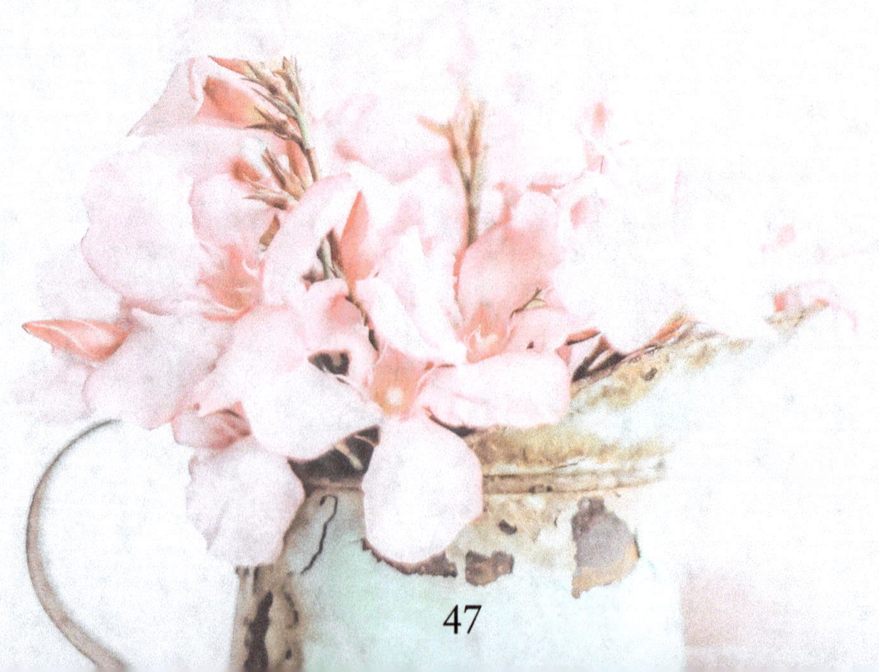

spring DIFFUSER BLENDS

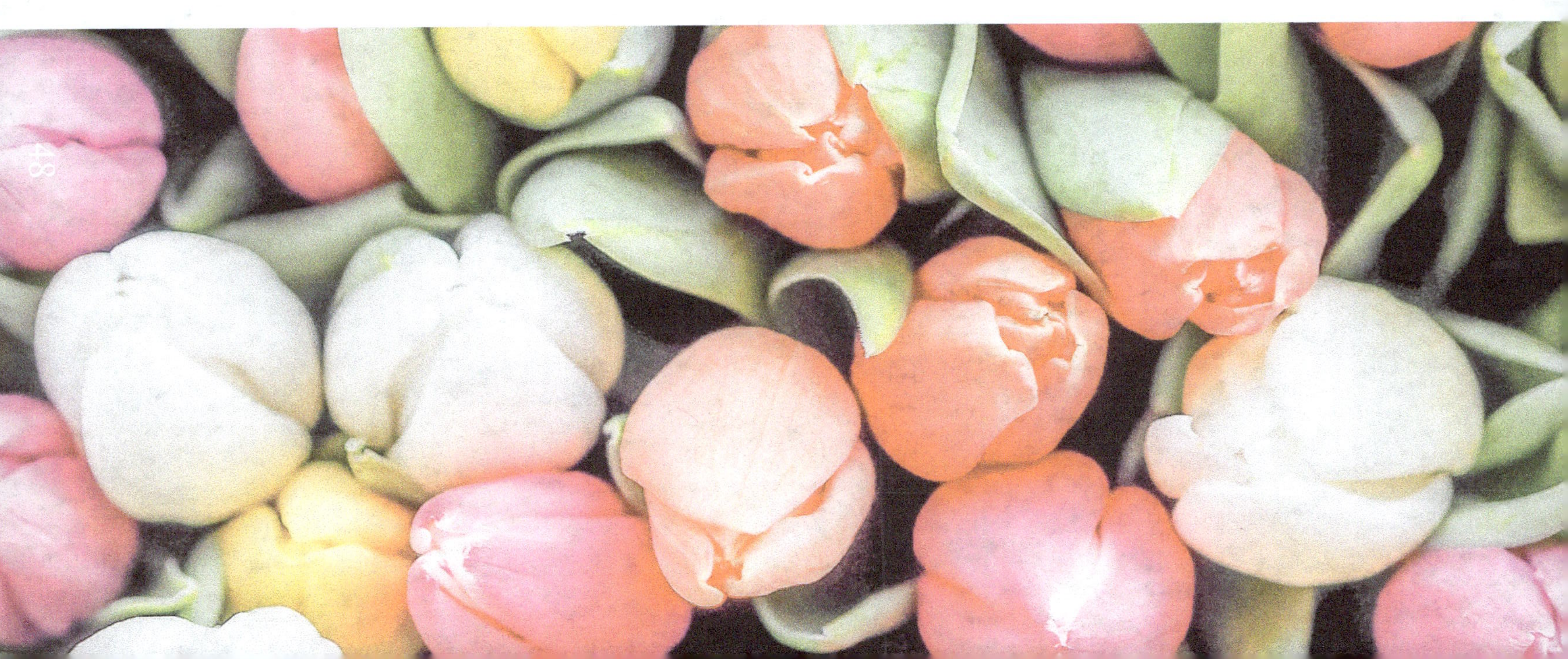

springtime

2 DROPS LIME
2 DROPS LAVENDER
2 DROPS WILD ORANGE

flower bliss

2 DROPS GERANIUM
2 DROPS GRAPEFRUIT
2 DROPS LEMON

sunshine

3 DROPS LEMON
2 DROPS BERGAMOT
2 DROPS LAVENDER

spring rain

2 DROPS LAVENDER
2 DROPS GERANIUM
2 DROPS CLARY SAGE

bliss

3 DROPS ROSE
2 DROPS BERGAMOT
2 DROPS LAVENDER

spring blooms

2 DROPS LIME
2 DROPS LAVENDER
2 DROPS WILD ORANGE

spring breeze

3 DROPS BERGAMOT
2 DROPS CEDARWOOD
2 DROPS YLANG YLANG

blooming flowers

2 DROPS LAVENDER
2 DROPS GERANIUM
2 DROPS CLARY SAGE

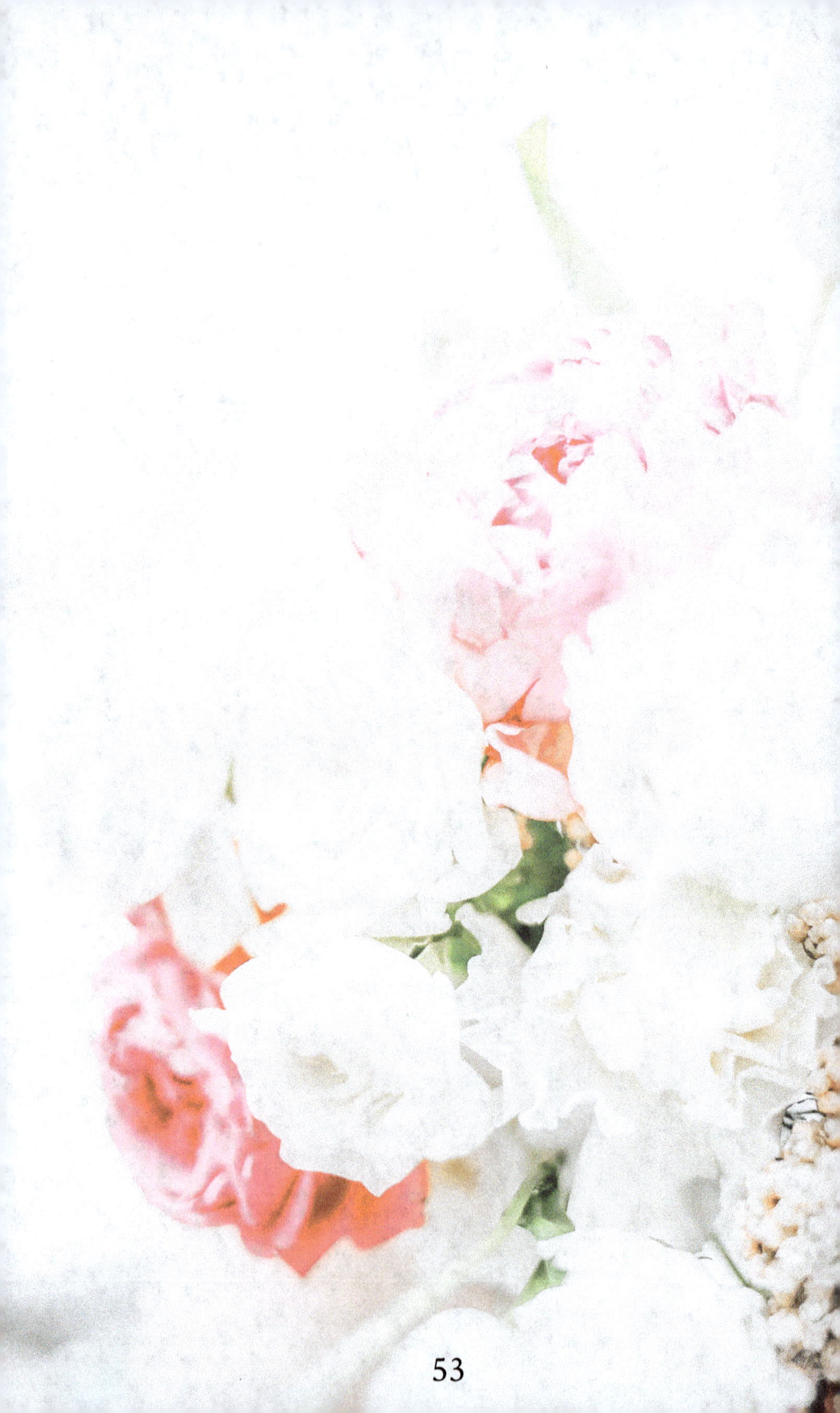

springtime bliss

2 DROPS WILD ORANGE
2 DROPS FRANKINCENSE
2 DROPS LIME

spring clean

3 DROPS LEMON
2 DROPS PEPPERMINT
2 DROPS LAVENDER

summer DIFFUSER BLENDS

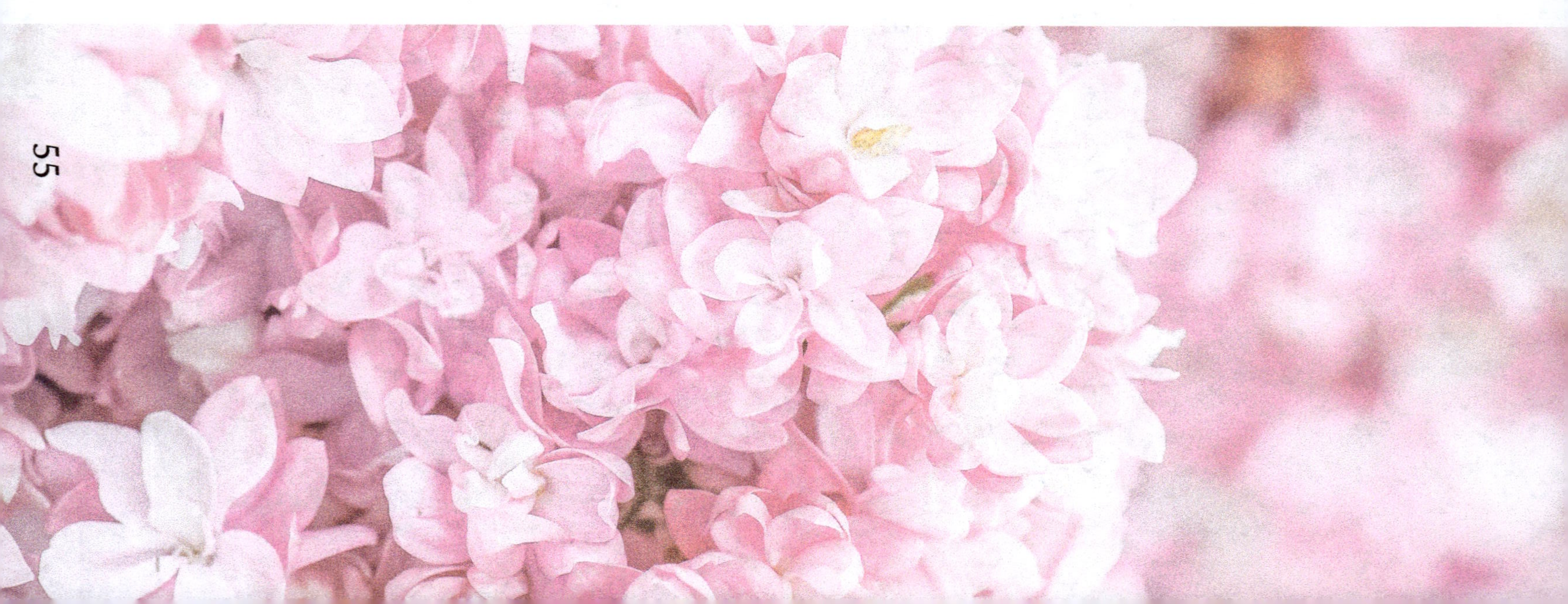

summer bliss

2 DROPS LEMON
2 DROPS BERGAMOT
2 DROPS TANGERINE

summer mornings

3 DROPS BERGAMOT
3 DROPS PEPPERMINT

citrus splash

2 DROPS GRAPEFRUIT
2 DROPS LIME
2 DROPS LEMON

beach vibes

2 DROPS SPEARMINT
2 DROPS LIME
2 DROPS TANGERINE

happy vibes

3 DROPS BERGAMOT
2 DROPS GRAPEFRUIT
2 DROPS WILD ORANGE

fresh air

2 DROPS EUCALYPTUS
2 DROPS LEMON
2 DROPS LAVENDER

beach waves

2 DROPS SPEARMINT
3 DROPS TANGERINE
2 DROPS BERGAMOT

flower bliss

2 DROPS LAVENDER
2 DROPS LEMON
2 DROPS GERANIUM
2 DROPS BERGAMOT

kids
DIFFUSER BLENDS

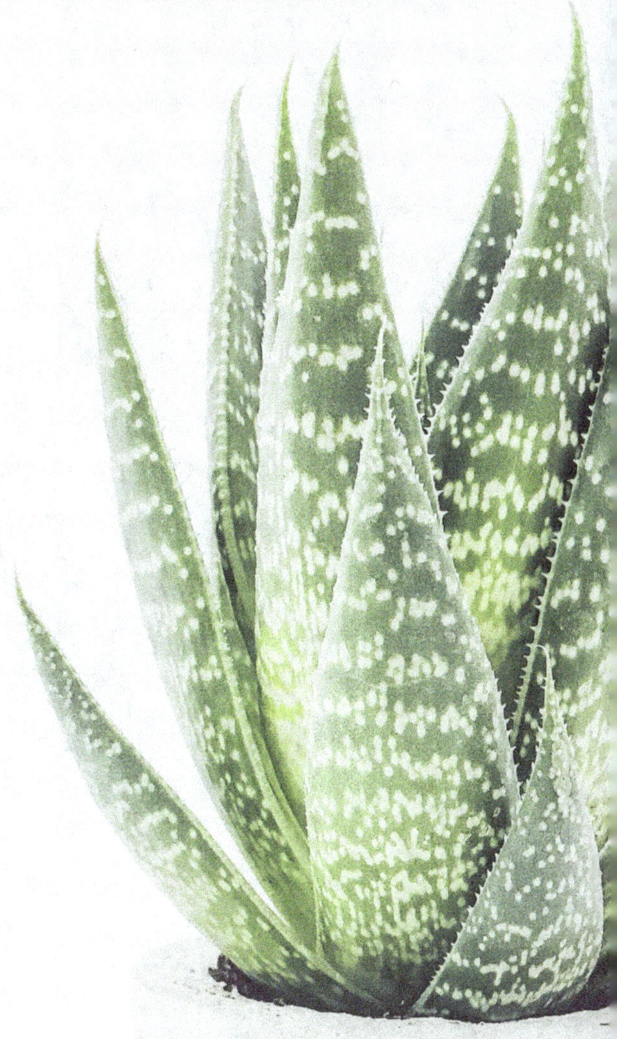

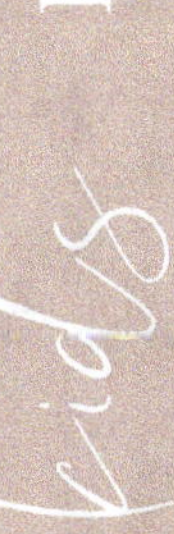

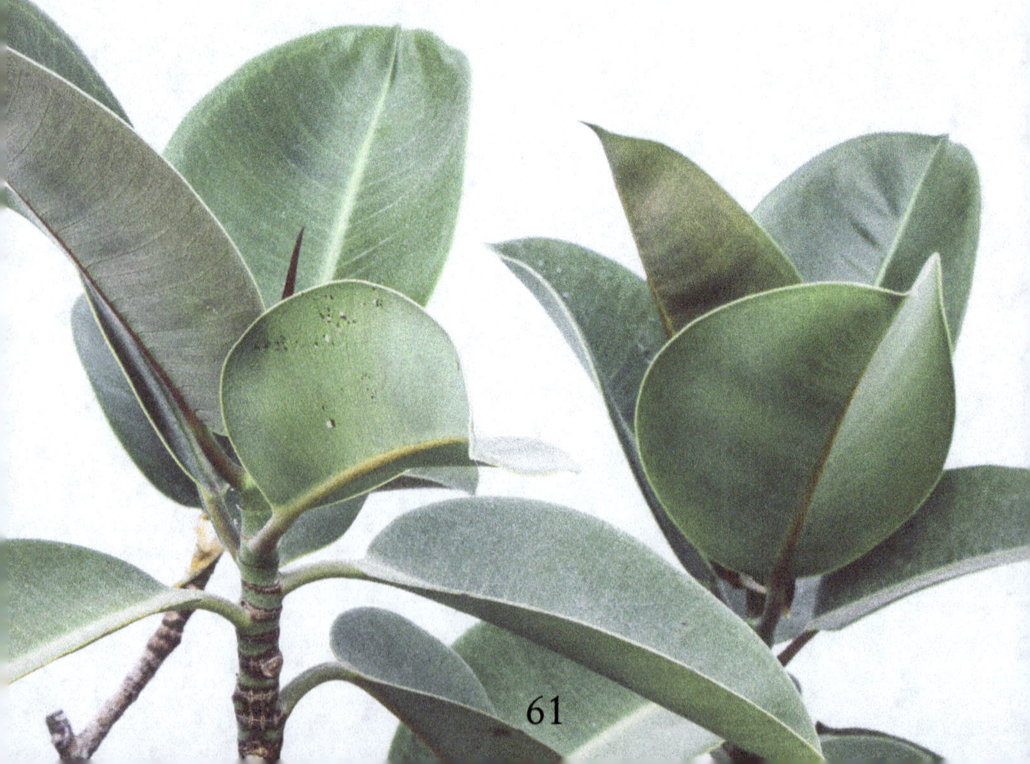

happy day

2 DROPS BERGAMOT
3 DROPS WILD ORANGE

study time

2 DROPS VETIVER
3 DROPS FRANKINCENSE

playroom

3 DROPS WILD ORANGE
3 DROPS LAVENDER

calming

3 DROPS CEDARWOOD
2 DROPS LAVENDER

night time

3 DROPS LAVENDER
3 DROPS VETIVER

good night

2 DROPS VETIVER
2 DROPS CEDARWOOD
2 DROPS JUNIPER BERRY

immune support

2 DROPS FRANKINCENSE
2 DROPS TEA TREE
2 DROPS LEMON

fresh air

3 DROPS LEMON
3 DROPS BERGAMOT

homework time

2 DROPS VETIVER
2 DROPS WILD ORANGE
1 DROP FRANKINCENSE

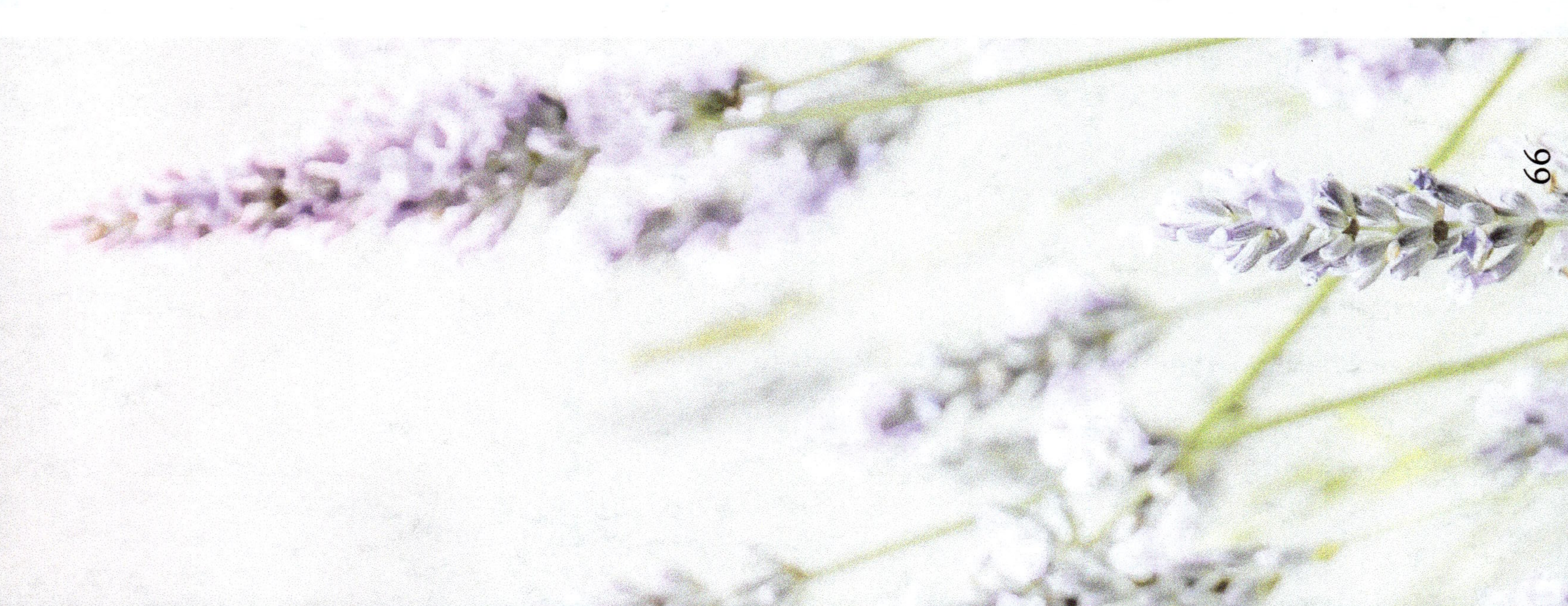

Lavender DIFFUSER BLENDS

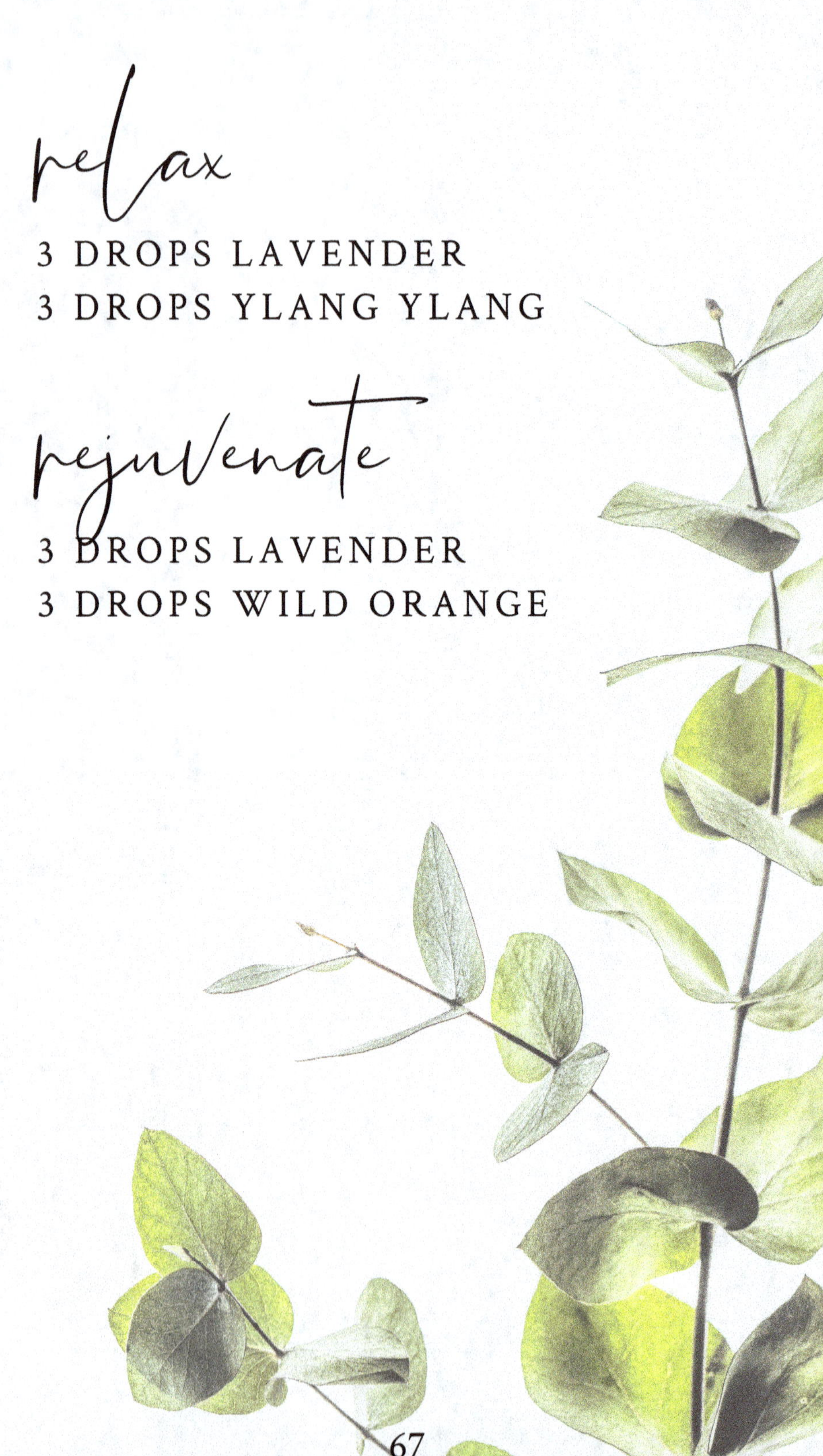

relax

3 DROPS LAVENDER
3 DROPS YLANG YLANG

rejuvenate

3 DROPS LAVENDER
3 DROPS WILD ORANGE

long day

2 DROPS LAVENDER
2 DROPS ROSEMARY
2 DROPS LEMON

sunset

3 DROPS LAVENDER
3 DROPS CEDARWOOD

sunshine

3 DROPS LEMON
2 DROPS BERGAMOT
2 DROPS LAVENDER

bliss

3 DROPS ROSE
2 DROPS BERGAMOT
2 DROPS LAVENDER

gentle

3 DROPS LAVENDER
3 DROPS FRANKINCENSE

lavender bliss

3 DROPS LAVENDER
2 DROPS BERGAMOT
2 DROPS CLARY SAGE

clean air

3 DROPS LEMON
3 DROPS LAVENDER

resources:

FIND MORE GREAT RECIPES
& NON-TOXIC LIVING TIPS AT
SIMPLYREENI.COM

GET ACCESS TO THE
FREEBIE LIBRARY AT
SIMPLYREENI.COM/FREE

SHOP OTHER
BEST-SELLING
RECIPE GUIDES &
COURSES AT
SHOPSIMPLYREENI.COM

Reeni is a Certified Essential Oils Coach, healthy living educator, author, and mom whose mission is to help women learn how to live their best lives naturally!

She started her business in 2016 as a blog to help others, and it's quickly grown into a thriving community and business! Reeni has many online healthy living guides and teaches online courses.

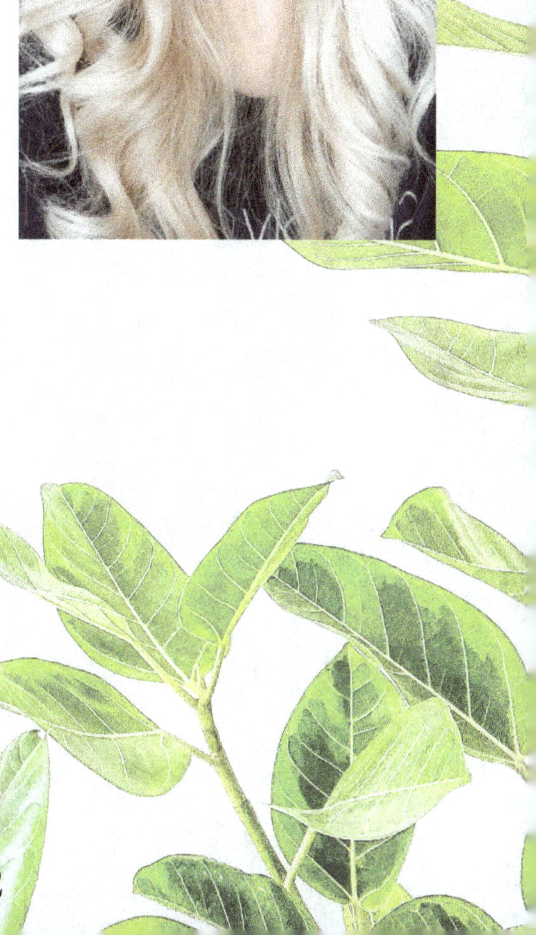